BAD MEMORY? WHAT IS IT AND HOW TO FIX IT?
15 TIPS FOR MEMORY IMPROVEMENT

Nancy Logan

COPYRIGHT

☐

Table of Contents

INTRODUCTION

In one sentence memory is basically the ability to store information to be retrieved at a later time. This can be information that you have learned for educational purposes, interesting facts, jokes or events that you need to remember. The things that you remember can be remembered on a short term or long term basis, depending on what type of information you are processing.

Short Term Memory

Short term memory comes in handy when you need to remember a number to dial, or an internet address, as your brain is designed to remember on average up to 7 items at a time. However, short term memory is not stored in your brain, and therefore as soon as you are done with it, it leaves your mind, and you cannot retrieve it later.

Long Term Memory

Long term memory on the other hand is stored in your brain so that you can retrieve it later when you need the information. This is information that you will need for a test, information to do your job, or information about family members, friends or events that you do not want to forget.

☐

HOW MEMORY WORKS

It sounds very simple, but the process of storing and retrieving information involves many parts of your brain. Some of the parts involved are the hippocampus, amygdala and cerebral cortex.

The ability to move information around depends on chemicals known as neurotransmitters. The neurons communicate with each other, and when new information enters, these neurons pass the information along and store it in the proper place in the brain.

But in order for the new information to be stored you need to concentrate on a single piece of information for up to 8 seconds. If you do not concentrate on the new information for this long, your brain will not be able to process and store this new information to be retrieved later. Therefore when you are trying to learn something new you should avoid multitasking, as it will hinder your ability to process new information.

Retrieving Information

After you have stored new information, your brain needs to activate the same path it took when it stored the information in your brain. This is why it helps you to repeat what you have learned as it helps your brain to remember the path more easily.

The more you use your memory, the stronger it will become allowing you to remember things in a short period of time, which you might never have thought to be possible.

Benefits Of A Good Memory

The present trends and happenings in life require that you need to be aware of memory improvement because you are required to remember a lot of things. Even you may be among the people who do not have a very good memory, and are likely to forget something or the other during your daily routine.

If this is the case, then you are also in the need of memory improvement. This is not a very worrying problem and there are methods for improving memory that can help. There are many such methods that can help you to get a better memory.

It is always best to look around and inform yourself of memory improvement methods and combine them so that you can take advantage of each of them. This can help you to gain a level of memory that can be very beneficial. Memory improvement can help you to improve the possibilities of your using increased memory.

Enhanced memory can lead to a number of benefits. You can then easily commit to mind the names of the people that you are constantly meeting in your day to day social interaction. This is especially beneficial if you do have to meet a lot of people during your daily job routines.

This will help you to impress people that you deal with and if they are clients, they will be satisfied enough to return to you time and again.

If you are working for a company, this fact can help you to be more productive in your job. This memory improvement would also enable you to remember a lot of numbers, something that is very much part of a daily routine nowadays.

There are telephone numbers to remember as are bank account numbers, identification numbers, credit card numbers and the like. In cases of emergency remembering the telephone numbers of your nearest and dearest can be a big advantage.

In the unlikely scenario, that you are in an accident, remembering telephone or contact numbers of your next of kin or even your medical practitioner can make your memory improvement the reason for your coming out of the trauma easily.

As a public speaker, an enhanced memory can help you to become a more effective speaker who can speak ex tempore instead of referring to written notes. This can be really impressive when you are called on without having any previous inkling that you would be re□uired to speak.

Public speakers would generally have lecterns in front of them where they can keep their prepared speeches and read from them. They could do with a course in memory improvement which would enable them to be far more effective speakers and speak from memory of points they remember from the notes they have made for the occasion.

There are other benefits that can accrue from memory improvement. You can remember very vividly reports you have read or seen on the electronic media of events that are in the current mind. So you can easily give your point of view when the same topics arise in a conversation and would easily be able to hold the attention of the people around you.

All these reasons are sufficient enough for a normal person to look for ways and means to go in for memory improvement for his or her memory.

□

TOP CAUSES OF MEMORY LOSS

When we talk about memory loss causes, we're simply talking about things that block you from being able to use your brain to its full extent.

Also, it's worth bearing in mind that if you tell yourself that you're losing your memory, you'll actually become more forgetful, which is the reason that the first in my list of memory loss causes is:

1. Telling Yourself You're Losing Your Memory

The human brain is an incredibly powerful tool. Its power to visualise in great detail, using all of your senses, is unrivalled and une☐ualled by even the most complex computers.

There are massive benefits to owning this supercomputer ability. Without going all metaphysical on you, it's possible to clearly visualise a chosen outcome and then allow your subconscious to come up with ways to make it happen.

The downside is that anything you've consistently told yourself - such as 'I'm losing my memory' - becomes fact in your subconscious. Regardless of whether it's a good or bad thing that you're telling yourself, from then on, your subconscious will work on the basis that you're right.

This can be catastrophic for your memory because your subconscious is working 24 hours per day, 365 days per year, even when you're asleep.

Think of it like a person constantly telling you that you're an idiot. Eventually, you might just start to believe it.

Solution:

Stop telling yourself you're losing your memory! - We all have memory gaps every so often, but they're not caused by 'losing' your memory. They may, in fact, be caused by some of the following factors...

2. Not Getting Enough Sleep

Another one of the major memory loss causes is sleep deprivation.

Your brain requires a certain amount of sleep per 24-hour cycle. Without it, your brain will be sluggish because it won't have the energy or rest time it needs to repair your body and mind after a day's work.

Significantly, with many of your functions impaired, you won't remember much. This is why staying up to study something the night before an exam is not a very bright thing to do.

Solution:

Get enough sleep! - This will vary slightly from person to person, but it's between 7.5 and 9 hours per 24-hour cycle for the majority of adults.

3. Stressing Your Mind

What if someone told you that you had to remember your full bank details in the next 20 seconds or you'll lose all your money?

How easy do you reckon it would be to remember any of it?

My guess? Not easy at all. The high stress and adrenalin levels in your brain would cause you to forget details because you'd be too focused on the time limit hanging over you and the potential loss of cash.

That's an extreme example, but the truth is, you're putting yourself under similar pressures all the time.

Stress is one of the biggest killers as it causes untold damage to your body. I'm talking about strokes, heart failure, the lot. It will also kill your memory.

Stress produces a hormone called cortisol which is damaging to the brain.
Many people would say that negative stress is unavoidable.

Regardless of what you think, there are ways to deal with stress that will help you to not be as affected by it. As a result of removing stress from the memory equation, you will remember more.

Solution:

Get some exercise - Regular exercise produces endorphins in your body which relax you and make you feel good, making it easier to remember.

Meditate - This allows your subconscious and conscious minds to interact more freely and removes tension by allowing you to be there, in that moment, without stress or anxiety. It's a lot harder than you might think to achieve that state, but when you do, it will open your mind to more learning.

Avoid prolonged high-stress activities - As an extreme example, if your job is to save people's lives (you might be a fireman or a surgeon), make sure you get the breaks you need between calls/operations and use them to do something that relaxes you.

4. Consuming a Poor Diet

I've spoken of this in other posts like this one, so here I want to focus on some specific elements that might be killing off your memory.

A balanced diet will allow your brain to get all the nutrients it needs to function.

Having a diet that's high in sugar, high in salt or full of additives (such as aspartame and monosodium glutamate) will damage your body as a whole and with regards to memory loss, damage your brain functions.

Solution:

Eat better (this really isn't rocket science, is it?) - Make sure you have three meals per day, with each one containing protein, fruit and/or vegetables and a complex carbohydrate. For example, bacon on wholegrain bread/toast with a glass of fruit smoothie for breakfast.

Don't snack on crap food that's high in sugar or salt, or that contains loads of additives.

Get plenty of water throughout the day. Dehydration will ruin your chance of functioning in a lot of areas, including memory.

5. Alcohol and Drug Use

This is pretty obvious, but I'm going to say it anyway as you may not realise the damage you're doing to yourself...
Drugs and alcohol (which is technically a drug too) can have negative effects on you for days after you consume them.
Sure, they may make you feel chilled out and at one with the world and your friends, but the fact is, they are damaging your brain.

According to Dr. John B. Arden, people who regularly consume alcohol display:

• Decreased performance on memory tests
• Decreased visual and spatial learning ability
• Decreased ability to make precise motor movements (their co-ordination is affected)
• Decreased short-term memory

And the list goes on and on...

Marijuana users tell a similar story.
Smoking pot regularly can make you irritable and lacking in motivation or clarity of thought.
Also, it is very well-known for causing significant short-term memory loss. If you smoke weed, your memories can become clouded and confused.

Solution:
Stop smoking pot - Seriously, I don't care how relaxed it makes you feel, it's damaging your memory in a BIG way. Unless you're being prescribed it because you have cancer or glaucoma, forget it. And even in those cases, it won't stop your memory from being affected.

Moderate your alcohol intake - The ideal situation is not to drink, but that's unrealistic. I like a glass of wine or a cheeky G&T as much as anyone. A little alcohol is OK, but excessive drinking or binging is just stupid.
Of course, there are other elements in your every day life that may be causing you to lose your memory.
One way to ensure they don't is to put into practice some of the top memory power tips, so that you can control and improve your memory power.

NUTRITION FOR MEMORY IMPROVEMENT

Just like nutritional diet helps us to have a healthy body, it helps in memory improvement as well. In our everyday life, there are several elements like stress, anxiety, lack of sleep, depression, and hormonal imbalances, which can adversely affect our mind and health. All these factors can lead to poor concentration, deteriorating skill and ability, as well as poor learning power, which are major signs of poor memory. However, the good news is that along with some other tips for improvement in memory, following nutritional diets can help you combat this situation.

There are a number of vitamins and minerals that help in memory improvement substantially. Here are the details -

Vitamin A helps in fighting the harmful toxins that can damage brain cells.

Vitamin B1 and Pantothenic Acid help in the production of acetylcholine, a brain cell chemical, which helps in improving concentration levels.

Vitamin B3 helps in overall brain health while B6 helps in improving the nerve communication.

Vitamin B12 plays a very important role in speeding up the electrical transmission rate in nerves by helping in the creation of myelin sheath for nerve protection.

Folic acid helps in guarding against the chance of Alzheimer's disease.

Vitamin C helps in destroying the free radicals, which may harm the brain cells.

Vitamin E helps in the overall functioning of your brain.

Selenium enhances the action of Vitamin E.

Zinc helps in memory improvement while iron boosts concentration.

The food we eat may not contain enough vitamins to sustain a healthy brain. Vitamin supplementation can compensate for this lack of nutrition and help with how to improve your memory. While all vitamins are important, some of them play special roles in memory improvement and you need them most if you have a sluggish memory.

Vitamin E. Best known for its antioxidant property, vitamin E prevents nerve damage in your brain due to lack of oxygen. The vitamin also prevents age-related memory loss. Furthermore, vitamin E has been proven to improve memory among the elderly. Other studies show it prevents Alzheimer's disease and that it delays its advancement in people who already suffer from it. Numerous foods provide vitamin E. Nuts, seeds, and vegetable oils are among the best sources of alpha-tocopherol, and significant amounts are available in green leafy vegetables and fortified cereals

Vitamin B6. It helps with how to improve your memory with continued supplementation. Vitamin B6 also speeds up the brain's capacity to store information as well as its ability to retain them. The richest sources of vitamin B6 include fish, beef liver and other organ meats, potatoes and other starchy vegetables, and fruit (other than citrus).

Vitamin B9. Also known as folic acid, this vitamin promotes the production of red blood cells which are responsible for bringing oxygen and nutrients to the brain. Folic acid also decreases the rate at which memory loss occurs. Good sources of B9 include broccoli, Brussels sprouts, asparagus and peas.

Vitamin B12. It works in a different way compared to vitamins B6 and B9. Unlike them, this vitamin decreases homocysteine levels. Homocysteine amino acids have been linked to poor brain functioning. Vitamin B12 also has this uni☐ue ability to repair damaged nerve fibers. It is best paired with vitamin B6 if you're wondering about how to improve your memory. Vitamin B12 is naturally found in animal products, including fish, meat, poultry, eggs, milk, and milk products.

Vitamin C. It is also an antioxidant like vitamin E. Thus, it can protect you from memory loss due to old age and other reasons. Vitamin C is available in abundance in many natural sources, including fresh fruits and vegetables. Eat your fruits and veggies raw whenever possible.

Vitamin D. Lack thereof prevents your brain from forming new memories. In the elderly, vitamin D deficiency is linked to memory loss. Supplementation should help alleviate these problems and help you how to improve your memory. The best food sources of vitamin D are fatty fish like salmon, herring and mackerel, and eggs.

A balanced meal of fruits, vegetables and nutritious food is your sure fire means to maintain a sharp memory. There are different benefits you can experience from eating the right food to offer you the nutrients you need, just spend time researching.

Other Supplements for Memory Improvement

There are several other health and nutritional supplements that can help a lot in your memory improvement endeavor. Take a look:

Apple Juice - Recent studies have shown that apple juice can help in the prevention of Alzheimer's diseases, which is associated with age related memory loss.

Fish and Fish Oils - DMAE, a very important chemical that is generally found in fish helps in the production of acetylcholine, which helps in improving concentration.

Apart from these, the consumption of fresh vegetables, fruits and low fat dairy products can also help in memory improvement. All these factors can lead to poor concentration, deteriorating skill and ability, as well as poor learning power, which are major signs of poor memory. However, the good news is that along with some other memory improvement tips, nutritional diets can help you combat this situation.Just like nutritional diet helps us to have a healthy body, it helps in memory improvement as well.

☐

15 TIPS FOR MEMORY IMPROVEMENT

Remembering is one significant skill in any individual that needs to be always honed and sharpened. With a good memory, you are always able to remember things like dates, names, currency figures and many other finer details. However, a poor remembrance habit is normally embarrassing especially in public and can lead to situations like low self-esteem. Therefore, you always need to look for ways in which you can enhance your memory so that you can avoid such life-dreaded circumstances. On that note, in the following discussion, we are going to look at 15 tricks to improve your memory.

1. Eat Right and Be Healthy

Our modern lifestyle has a few adverse effects on the power of our memories. From food habits to enormous stress and avoiding proper rest - all these play detrimental roles to improving memory. This is the reason it is of paramount importance to lead a healthy life with quality food habits.

It's on record that eating foods and supplements that contain flavonoids such as berries, grapes, tea leaves, hops, cocoa beans greatly boosts the neurons in the brain in the sense that they are able to form fresh memories. Additionally, these foods normally associate with enzymes and proteins that are significant for the memory and, even more importantly, help in the formation of new neurons and the crucially sufficient flow of oxygen into the brain. The anti-inflammatory and antioxidant properties of vitamin D helps to maintain healthy brain functions.

So, if you are keen to develop your memory, you must restrain yourself from junk foods and alcohol. Moreover, just like the body, the brain also needs sound rest to work at its utmost potential. As far as foods are concerned, you need to include fruits and green vegetables in your daily diet that supply the needed antioxidants to protect the brain cells from getting damaged.

2. Avoid Sugar

Sweet dishes are common weakness for many and if you are one of them, you may find it sad to know that intaking refined sugar more than the recommended limit can be harmful for your memory. Let's find out how sugar can affect the memory.

There is a significant amount of data to indicate that a high intake of refined sugar into the body of a human being has a detrimental effect on the brain and memory health. Many people consume in a day about double the amount of sugar calories recommended by the medical experts. Refined sugar leads to difficulties in forming new memories, depression, and a reduction in the brain functions. Refined sugar minimizes the production of Brain-Derived Neurotrophic Factor (BDNF) which is a very crucial element when it comes to learning and creating new memories.

3. Drink Caffeine

Caffeine has a positive effect on the memory relative to taking other substances. However, this must be done carefully to avoid habitual consumption. After consuming coffee, several cognitive tasks are carried out and in the final analyses drinking caffeine enhances the memory of a human being.

Adding to that, green tea also has a very positive role to play when it comes to improving the memory. It contains polyphenols, a powerful antioxidant that prevents free radicals from damaging the brain cells. Moreover, regular consumption of green tea is the best guide to improve memory and mental alertness and it can significantly slow the brain-aging process.

4. Exercise Your Brain

Appropriate brain exercises can help keeping your brain active through ages. Just like the muscles of the body, our brain, too, needs food and exercise of its own type. There are certain exercises that help in evolving the functionality of the brain and the power of memory. You can consider them as these are the best memory improving tricks. Moreover, if you keep on practicing these exercises over a long period of time, it's going to bring some miraculous results for you.

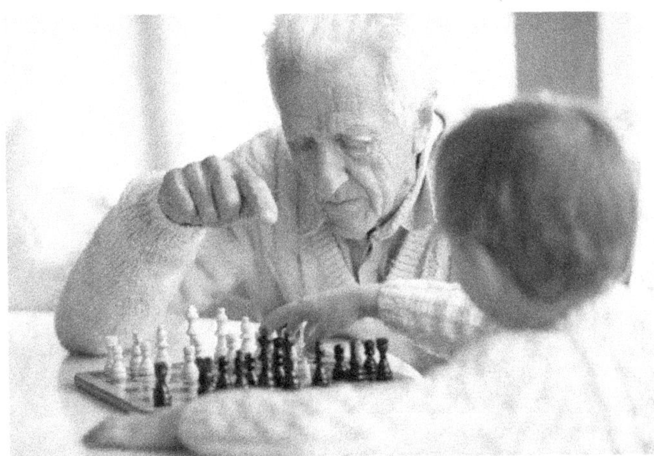

There are several ways in which you can exercise your brain to improve it. Some of these include reading as much as you can, increasing your vocabulary, learning new languages, writing something, post problem solving and turning off the television. You can also play games such as chess, cards or even solve puzzles. With these activities you can exercise your brain and, more importantly, expand your memory, thus improving it.

5. Exercise Daily

It is said that "to achieve something you never had, you must do something you never did".

In today's busy world health is the most neglected aspect of our lives whereas, it should be the other way around! We must manage at least half an hour everyday to devote to our health. Daily exercise has multiple physical and mental benefits to offer and undoubtedly, when it's about improving the memory power, one can receive splendid results through this process.

Daily

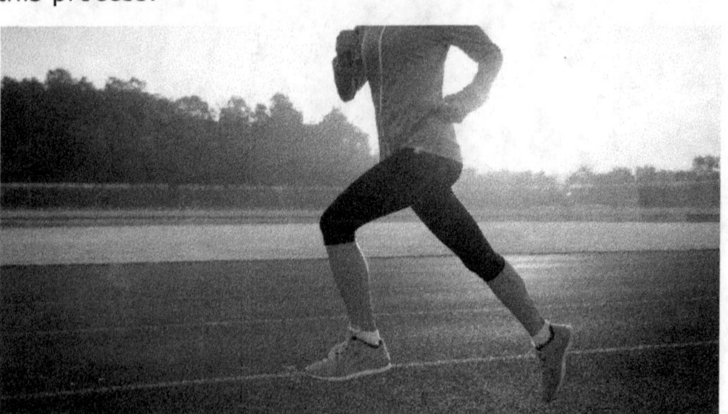

exercise can immensely enhance your brain and thinking skills. This is achieved through indirect and direct means. Through direct means, it acts on the body by stimulating physiological changes such as inflammation and reductions in insulin resistance as well as encouraging production of growth factors. It directly works on your brain by improving your sleep and mood. Through this, it's crystal-clear that consistent daily exercise is a great recipe for the improvement of your memory.

6. No Multitasking

It sounds great to have a title of "multitasking" but, do you want to know that what type of impact it has on your brain? While we are discussing about how to improve the brain's memory, you may get disappointed to know that multitasking is not helpful in improving your brain's memory.

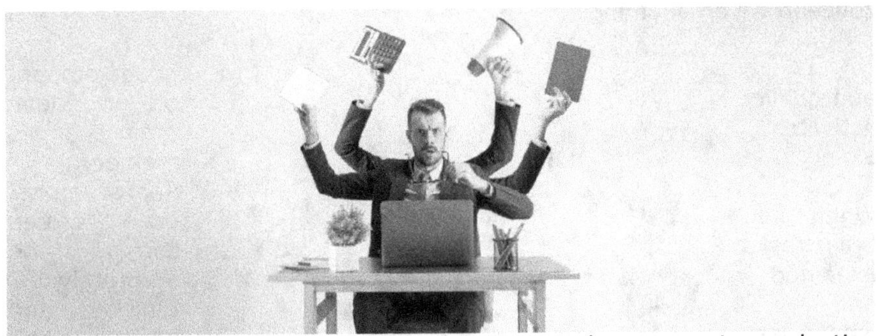

Many times, multitasking has been termed as a counterproductive and exhaustive process. An average and perfectly working mind prefers shifting from one task to another instead of multitasking. Therefore, the exhaustive nature of multitasking, does not in anyway, improve the nature of your memory.

Various studies have already suggested that it not just causes a lack of concentration, it might slow down the work process and cause errors! If you are trying to complete 3-4 tasks by a certain point of time, you better put attention on the individual tasks because it will take much less time to complete than all the tasks being performed together. This is why it is one of the best tips to improving memory.

7. Sleep Well

After a long day of work, our body needs sound sleep at night and this is also important to stabilize the functionality of the brain. The brain performs thousands of activities throughout the day and a good sleep of 6-8 hours stabilizes the brain and puts it into the best working condition the next morning. On the contrary, not having proper sleep in the night will make you drowsy for the entire day and you will not be able to concentrate on anything.

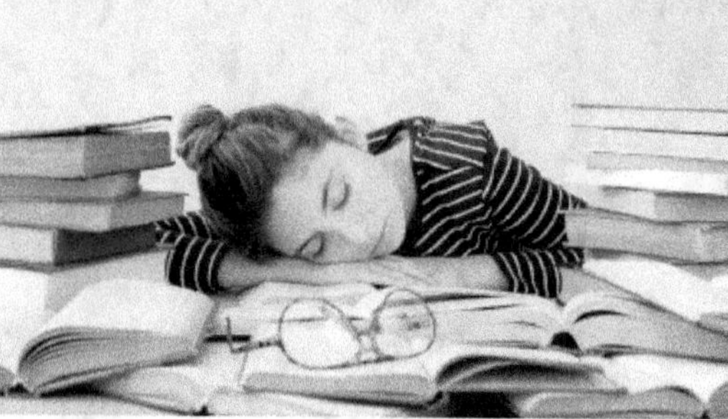

A good amount and quality of sleep activates brain changes aiding in memory improvement. When you are asleep brain tasks can be executed accurately and Quickly with less anxiety and pressure. This is basically a recipe for boosting the capacity of your memory.

A study conducted amongst children suggests that when kids take naps between learning lessons and testing them in real life, they are very likely to perform better. It helps the process of brain growth (called neuroplasticity) that controls the brain's capacity to control behavior of learning and memory. So, sleeping well is very much associated with the brain's memory improvement.

8. Reduce Stress and Laugh More

Stress and depression can actually take a toll on one's ability to remember things. However, by engaging yourself in laughter, you reduce the levels of your stress and improve the capabilities of your memory. In a nutshell, laughter brings down the cortisol stress hormone.

Sometimes, we put so much stress on ourselves without even realizing the bad impact that it is having on our health and brain. It puts way more pressure on the heart and when it comes to the brain, you experience a lack in its memory power. Laughter is indeed a great medicine to get rid of this situation! With the help of emotional responses, only a few parts of the brain are activated but, with laughter, all the regions of the brain are engaged. This is the reason, it is helpful to spend time with light-hearted people and laugh everyday as it is one of the proven tricks to boost your memory.

9. Chew Gum

Chewing gum helps to remember more. People who chew gum test both the short-term and long-term memory. These gum-chewers are deemed to produce higher scores than those who do not chew gum when it comes to remembering things. It is difficult to explain the scientific reasons behind this but, over time, it has shown some effective results for people who are keen to know "how can I improve my memory?"

10. Learn a New Skill

They say keeping your brain busy with learning new things has a good impact on improving your memories. This is also one of the best memory improvement tricks that everyone must apply. The question here is - does age have anything to do with this process. It is seen that keeping your brain busy with purposeful and meaningful activities improves the neurological system and this is how to boost your memory. Science has already proved that this has no relevance with age.

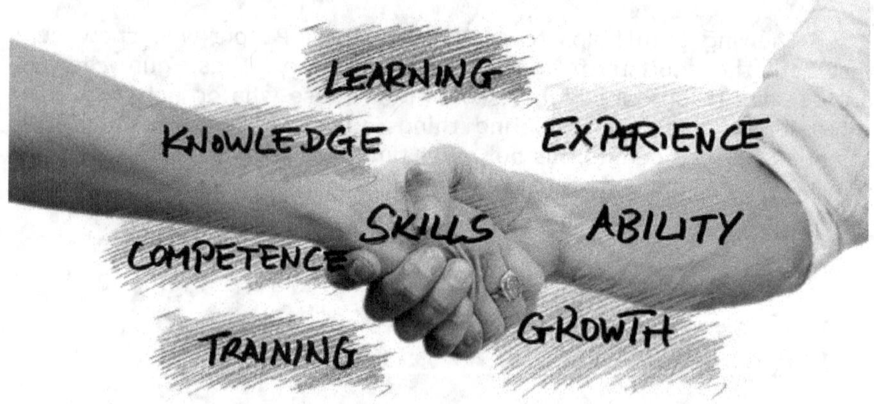

It's always been true that if you want to enhance your brain you must work on it. Learning a new skill that you were initially unfamiliar with has a significant effect on improving your brain. People who always engage their brains in learning new things always demonstrate improved memory function. As a person gets older, by trying new things, he/she ensures a healthy mind.

11. Try Mnemonic Devices

In our everyday life, we come across a lot of things and we can't really keep all of them in our memory. Probably, we don't want to store all of them in the memory. But, what about those incidents, names, events, dates that you want to keep in your memory but face challenges? You can simply try Mnemonic devices as one of the best tricks to boost your memory.

Mnemonic devices are basically memory techniues that aid the brain to encode better, and importantly, remember some fine, but important details. An example of a mnemonic device is the famous '30 days hath September' rhyme which is very significant in helping so many of us to remember how many days in each calendar month. Sometimes, without mnemonic devices, it's often harder to remember some things. Regarding new studies, these techniques highly improve the state of your memory.

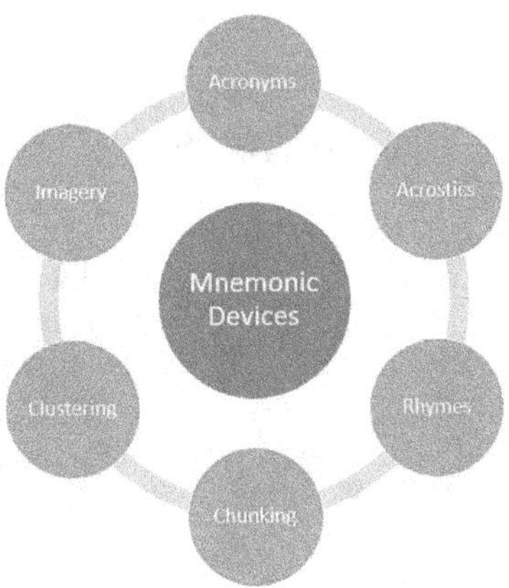

There are many other similar devices that you can be applied for this purpose but, the best thing you can do is to innovate some own techniues to improve memory. It works excellent!

12. Association

Every piece of information that we think of is always linked to another piece in one way or another. Our memory basically works by association. For better remembrance, we always try to create an association between pieces of information. When two bits of information are related to each other, we have a greater capability to be creative in linking the two and, as a result this enhances our memories.

13. Rhymes

This may sound like an old-school method, but sometimes, forming rhymes really help memorizing things much better. Our brain is not configured to remember multiple things at the same time but, forming those details in a rhyme structure is helpful to keep them in mind and apply at the right time. This is the best guide to improve memory. After practicing it for a particular time, it becomes very exciting for anyone to remember things in the form of rhymes.

It's always easier to forget a list of six items in a shopping list than it is to forget the lyrics of a song you have not heard for ages. Basically, our brains easily remember things by rhymes since they are linked to each other. Therefore, a person who knows a poem can more easily remember it than remembering random words. This is an excellent way in which you can enhance your brains since you can rhyme things making them exciting and memorable.

14. Flash Cards

Flashcards are commonly used in schools and institutions to help learn school subject material. With flashcards, you are able to remember things like vocabulary and □uestions about a subject. Flashcards re□uire you to take time so that you can make the studies more useful and memorizing more effective. Through the use of flashcards, you can greatly boost your memory.

How to make and use a flash cards?

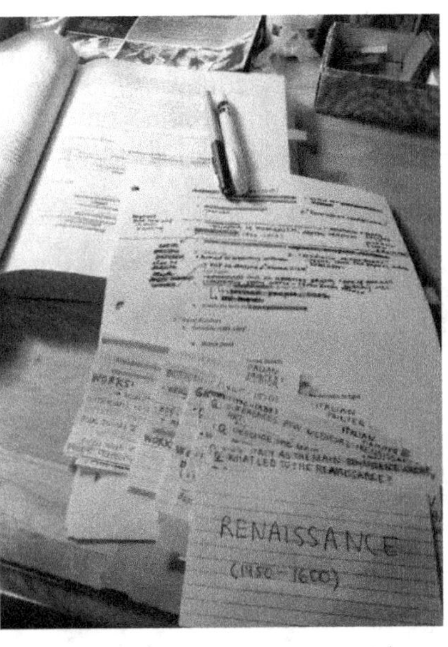

1. Take a paper and write a question on one side, and the right answer on the other side.
2. Read the question and try to answer correctly -
3. If you succeed to answer right, you put it aside, if you did not, you save it for latter.
4. You need to do this until you remember every single answer without looking.

15. Organize Your Life

This is an amazing fact to know that the first thing you do after lifting yourself up from the bed to the last thing you do before going to sleep has an impact on our memory. The more organized your life is, the better your memory will become. Your regular activities, food habits and even your sleeping habits - all these have significant impact on the memory.

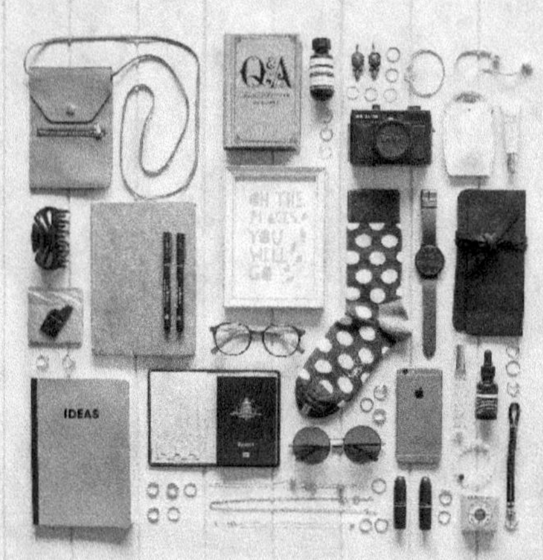

When your life is organized, it basically means you can distinctly identify one item you are doing from another. An organized life means that the brain works at a certain procedure. This becomes very important when it comes to remembering some things. Therefore, an organized life is a good recipe for an excellent memory capacity.

Moreover, when you do things in an organized way, the brain can also work in an organized manner and that is directly related to the improving of your memory.